BASIC ✶ ESSENTIALS

SURVIVAL

Help Us Keep This Guide Up to Date

Every effort has been made by the author and editors to make this guide as accurate and useful as possible. However, many things can change after a guide is published—new products and information become available, regulations change, techniques evolve, etc.

We would love to hear from you concerning your experience with this guide and how you feel it could be improved and be kept up to date. While we may not be able to respond to all comments and suggestions, we'll take them to heart and we'll also make certain to share them with the author. Please send your comments and suggestions to the following address:

The Globe Pequot Press
Reader Response/Editorial Department
P.O. Box 480
Guilford, CT 06437

Or you may e-mail us at:

editorial@globe-pequot.com

Thanks for your input.

BASIC ESSENTIALS™ SERIES

BASIC ✳ ESSENTIALS™

SURVIVAL

SECOND EDITION

BY JAMES CHURCHILL

The Globe Pequot Press

Guilford, Connecticut

Cover photo: Corel Images
Cover design by Lana Mullen
Text and layout design by Casey Shain
Illustrations: Figures 6, 10, 14, 15, 16, and 20 by Scott Power. Figures 8, 11, 12, 18, 24, 33, and 34 by Carole Drong.
Interior photographs by James Churchill

Library of Congress Cataloging-in-Publication Data is available.

ISBN: 0-7627-0525-6

Manufactured in the United States of America
Second Edition/First Printing

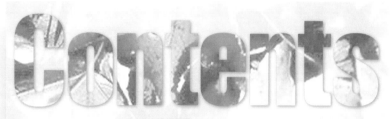

Introduction

This book is a basic guide to the skills you might need if suddenly stranded, whether in the deep wilderness or only a few miles from home. But, far more important than any book or device is your reasoning ability and attitude.

The Creator gave us the ability to overcome any challenge. But when faced with danger, we must stay calm and allow the reasoning process to develop. And never give up. Always keep trying. The worst challenge you will ever face has probably been overcome by someone before. People have endured incredible deprivation and lived to tell about it.

The object of this book is to outline the skills and tell what action you should take so you don't ever have to see how much misery you can endure. Never go into territory without knowing which way you must go to get out. Always carry a compass and learn how to use it. Always dress for the worst conditions you might encounter and carry a basic survival kit. Finally, make sure someone knows where you have gone so searchers know where to start looking for you.

Learn how to make a fire with natural materials and build a shelter from the forest or plains. Learn to catch animals, fish, and find edible wild plants, and prepare them.

Almost anything can be made from natural objects if you have the skill. I once watched John Sinclair make an excellent stone knife from the stones and shrubs growing around our cabin in northern Wisconsin. I am still using this stone knife years later for certain projects. If you develop your skills and knowledge beforehand, getting stranded may be more interesting than exhausting.

Also learn to utilize what you have along. For instance, a brightly colored sleeping bag waved aloft is a noticeable signaling device, and the cosmetic mirror you have along can be used to reflect sunlight into the cabin of an aircraft to alert the pilot.

Just for Kids

When you are camping or playing in wilderness areas, always wear a police whistle around your neck. If you can't see camp or other people, stay where you are and blow your whistle. If you get really lost and have to stay out overnight, curl up under a fallen tree or cover yourself with leaves. Next morning find an open space and stay in it so a helicopter can spot you. Continue to blow your whistle and shout. Make tracks in sand so that they can be seen. If you see strange people who shout your name, don't run away from them. They like you and want to take you back home again. Go up to them or blow your whistle.

The Globe Pequot Press assumes no liability for accidents happening to, or injuries sustained by, readers who engage in the activities described in this book.

Making a Fire

A brightly burning campfire is a source of warmth and light. It is a cheerful companion and confidence builder, and it can be used to signal help, acquire and cook food, sterilize water, repel dangerous wild animals, and shape natural objects into useful tools. (See Chapter 4 for more information on using fire to acquire food.) Making a fire should be the first order of business when lost or stranded.

In this modern age there are a great many people who have never built a fire at all, and a great many more who have never built one without fire-starting fluids. This is more difficult than might be realized and should be the first skill you acquire if you're going to be at risk of getting stranded in the backcountry. Practice building fires in widely different areas so you can learn to recognize burnable material. *Make very sure each fire is completely out before leaving it.*

No one should go into a wilderness area without some means of starting a fire. I carry a plastic 35mm film container full of stick matches. I have to break them off to fit, but this small container will hold two dozen matches if the ends are alternated. It can be carried in any pocket and will keep the matches dry even if I fall in the water. I have several of these containers, and recently discovered one that had been in a coat pocket for a year. The matches still worked perfectly.

Fire Starters

Place a small piece of emery cloth in the container to strike matches on. Take at least 200 matches; also take at least four candles along. Use a match to light the candle, then use the candle to light tinder to start a fire. Candles will also furnish light and can be used for light cooking. If you set the candle in a container, it can be recycled.

Waterproof camping matches are available from camping supply outlets, or you can make your own by coating kitchen matches with paraffin.

An excellent fire starter for survivors is a device called a magnesium fire starter or "metal match." It consists of a block of magnesium and a flint insert. A small pile of magnesium is scraped from the block with a knife. Then the insert is scraped with the knife to produce fat, hot sparks that will ignite the magnesium. This device will work even if it gets wet, and the burning magnesium will ignite any dry tinder. A disposable cigarette lighter is also a good fire starter, and most will give more than 1,000 lights. They are light in weight and inexpensive and will work even after they get wet.

Primitive Methods

People do get lost, however, and for one reason or another have no fire-making materials along, or they quickly use up their supply of matches. Therefore, every outdoorsperson should practice making a fire by primitive methods. If nothing else, finding out how demanding and time consuming starting a fire without matches is, will remind the traveler to carry a good supply of matches on every backcountry trip.

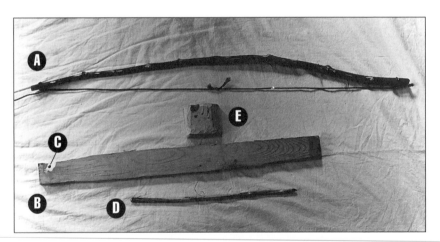

Figure 1

Bow and drill fire starter. The bow (A) should be 36" in length. The fire board (B) should be 30" in length. However, the fire hole (C) should be put in on the flat side about 24" from a chosen end. The drill (D) is 18" in length, and the socket (E), which holds the drill, is 3" in width.

The bow-and-drill method of starting a fire is the most versatile (see Figures 1 and 2). It should be learned by anyone who is at risk of getting lost or stranded. The raw materials are at hand wherever trees grow. The string for the bow can be made from a boot lace or even coated wire from a vehicle's wiring harness. This method is far from easy. Don't wait until you are stranded to learn how it's done.

I spent about eight hours of concentrated activity before getting a fire burning from a bow and drill. But now that the device is made, I can usually get a fire going in a half hour or so. A new hole has to be drilled in the fire board every two or three lights because the drill will wear out the original hole. The fire drill has to be reshaped quite often also.

Here's how I made mine: Using a large belt knife, I split a 3-foot length of white spruce limb to make the fire board. It is about 1 inch thick and 3 inches wide. Next I found a dead seasoned maple sapling about 5/8 inch in diameter and shaped it into a fire drill 18 inches long. The bottom end was tapered to about a 45 degree angle, and the top of the drill was simply rounded off and made as smooth as possible. The drill headpiece was a dead, seasoned piece of maple log about 3 inches square. A socket was gouged into the center of the headpiece to fit the top end of the drill. I lubricated it with earwax and oil from beside my nose.

Working carefully I used the point of the knife to drill a hole in the fire board that would fit the taper on the fire drill. Directly underneath the hole, a V-shaped notch was formed to hold the tinder.

A hard maple limb with a natural bow shape made a 36-inch-long bow. I used my boot laces for a bow string. Notches were cut near each end of the bow to keep the laces from slipping. The string has to be tied fairly snug but not too tight because the fire drill is wrapped in the string.

I placed the tapered point of the drill in the hole in the fire board, held the top with the headpiece, and sawed the bow back and forth to spin the drill. The drill soon milled the hole to a snug fit, and shortly thereafter smoke started coming from the hole. I stopped then and went looking for tinder.

I found a dead cedar tree and made tinder from the inner bark. I shredded it until it was so light and fluffy it would almost float in the air. I packed the tinder into the V notch under the hole in the fire board. Finally after several hours of drilling, reshaping the drill and its seat in the fire board, and trying again, I got the tinder smoldering and blew it into a flame.

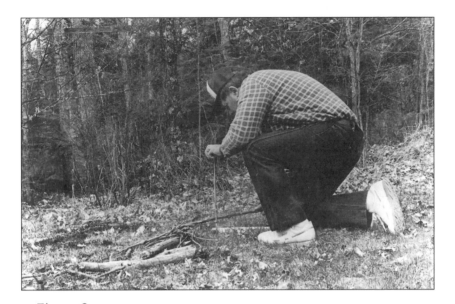

Figure 2

Make a fire using a bow and drill.

To sum up: This method of making a fire is far from easy or quick, but it definitely works. Best of all, the components can be built from natural materials, and if no knife is at hand, they probably could be made with a sharp rock or a piece of broken glass.

Using What's at Hand

If you have a black powder firearm along, you can sometimes start a fire by ramming tinder down the barrel against the powder charge. Use charred cloth if available. Fire the gun up in the air, run and pick up the cloth and blow it into flame. Have a supply of tinder at hand so that the cloth can be placed against it to start the fire.

Fires can be started with a magnifying glass if the sun is nearly overhead and shining brightly. You can carry a small magnifying glass along on an expedition for just this purpose. I have a "bull's-eye" magnifying glass that will start a fire in a minute or less when good tinder is available (see Figure 3). But with any type of magnifying glass, you have to move the lens back and forth until you've adjusted the sunlight shining through the glass to a small brilliant dot. Situate the dot to shine on a tight ball of tinder and it will quickly start smoking.

4   B A S I C   E S S E N T I A L S

Hold the tinder in one hand and the magnifying glass in the other so you can blow on the tinder after it starts smoldering. This is not as easy as it might sound, and you should practice this procedure before-hand.

A telephoto lens from a camera also can be used to start a fire (Figure 4). Remove the lens from the camera and use the same proce-dure as you did with the magnifying glass. Lenses taken from binocu-lars and telescopic rifle sights also can be put together to produce a magnifying glass to start a fire.

We have created fire with both smokeless and black powder, a tin can lid, and a magnifying glass. We shaped the lid to a bowl shape and fastened it on a stump so that it protruded over the edge to cut down on heat conduction. We filled the lid with powder and direct-ed the bull's-eye of light on the metal under the powder. In a few sec-onds to a few minutes, the powder would ignite with a noticeable "poof" into a significant flame.

Discarded bottles and decorative glass figurines have, reportedly, accidentally started fires that burned forests and dwellings by concen-trating the sun's rays on burnable material. If no magnifying glass is at hand, experiment with other materials.

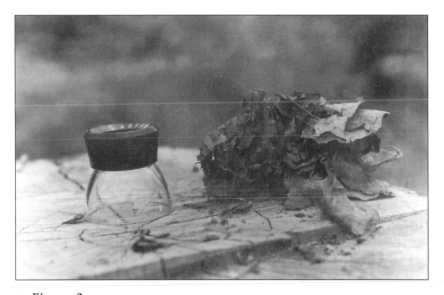

Figure 3

A bull's-eye magnifying glass and natural tinders will quickly start a fire.

If a vehicle, airplane, or boat motor that still runs is available, you can probably get a fire started by placing a rag or other tinder directly on the exhaust manifold. Soak the tinder with fuel if feasible. Start the engine and run it at high speed to make the manifold hot. Have a pile of tinder ready and transfer the burning rag to the tinder. If having a fire is more important than keeping the vehicle intact, you can definitely set it afire by loosening or cracking a fuel line in the right place so fuel drips on the exhaust manifold. Start the engine and let it run until it starts burning. This also will create a smoke signal for signaling rescuers.

A tire can probably be set afire by raising the vehicle so that the tire barely touches a log or rough rock. Place the vehicle in gear and spin the rubber tire against the friction of the log/rock until it starts burning.

A battery from a disabled vehicle or airplane can be used to quickly start a fire (Figure 5). Take it out of the vehicle if possible. Then tear out a two- to three-foot-long piece of wire from the vehicle's wiring harness. Use headlight wiring or some other noncritical wiring if the vehicle might be used again. Strip both ends of the wire and wrap one end around the negative terminal of the battery. Then find

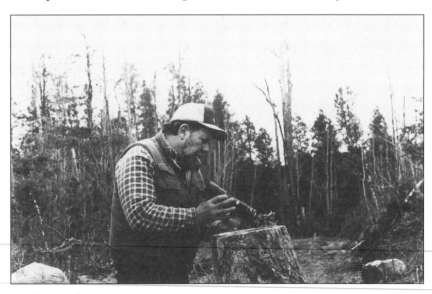

Figure 4

A telephoto lens and natural tinder will also start a fire.

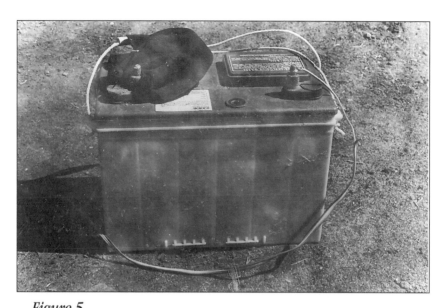

Figure 5
....

Start a fire with a battery and gasoline soaked rag. Use other tinder if no rags or gasoline are available.

a rag and soak it with gasoline. Loosen or break a fuel line if you can't dip the rag in the tank. Lay the gasoline soaked rag against the positive terminal. Then using gloves, touch the other end of the wire to the positive terminal. The rag will ignite instantly. Place the burning rag under some previously gathered tinder. No need to use fine tinder for this fire. Instead, good-sized dead twigs can be set afire.

Realize that there are some slight risks connected with this procedure. If the battery has vent holes in the caps, ignitable fumes might escape from the vent during this attempt, especially if you use large diameter wire to "short" across the battery terminal. The fumes might ignite, and there is a slight risk that the battery will explode. If your face is close to the battery, you could get sulfuric acid in your eyes, which could cause blindness. Eliminate the risk by using a long stick to place the wire against the positive terminal. Protect your eyes with whatever is at hand. This could range from looking through a piece of glass to making a bark mask with thin slits for eye holes, to standing behind a tree during actual contact. Immediately immerse in water body parts that become contaminated with sulfuric acid.

If sparks are the only way to get a fire started, try out, maybe after dark when sparks are easier to see, any metal or rocks at hand to see if they will produce a hot spark, as some will. Accidental fires have been started by a combination of volatile fuel and sparks from casually thrown rocks.

I have tried to get a fire burning without success from sparks made with flint and steel; from firing a gun fueled with smokeless, modern powder; with a fire plough; and with a fire thong. I don't believe they are workable ways for a survivor to get a fire burning, even though they are recommended in many books.

Tinder

Regardless of the method used for making a fire, however, it won't be successful without good tinder. Learn to recognize this material before you get stranded. Use the inner bark from dead trees, dry small twigs shredded between the fingers, dead grass shredded between the fingers, mouse nests, downy feathers, wasps nests, dried evergreen needles, dry moss, cattail fluff, punky material from inside dead elderberry stalks, and dried animal dung, which all make good tinder.

If the surrounding forest is wet, finding dry tinder is more difficult. Try the wispy bark from birch trees that can be gathered without a knife. It is impregnated with oil and doesn't absorb moisture. The inner bark from dead standing trees and the inner core of a rotting stump that can be kicked apart might have dry tinder. Don't forget that the paper in your wallet, the cuffs of your shirt, your handkerchief, or even the top of your shirt tail can be shredded to make tinder when the surrounding area is wet.

Firewood

Good tinder is very important to start the fire, but good dry fuel to keep it burning is equally as important. Be sure the fuel is piled so the tinder can be placed underneath it. Tiny dry twigs piled tepee fashion will quickly catch fire if placed over burning tinder. Have some larger twigs at hand to put on the fire. After branches an inch or so in diameter are burning, there will be time to gather larger pieces for fuel. Gradually increase the size until logs 6 inches or more in diameter will burn. They will hold a fire for hours. If they can't be cut up in short lengths, just push the ends into the fire, let them burn off, and push up another length.

Sometimes it is easier to make up fuzz sticks than to find small twigs. Take a short length of twig an inch or so in diameter and whittle it toward one end so a shaving is produced. But don't cut the shaving off. Leave it on the branch so that the end result looks like a shuttlecock. Lean the fuzz sticks against each other, tepee fashion, and place the burning tinder underneath them.

You will fuel most survival fires with whatever wood is nearby. Seldom will you have a choice of woods to use. Soft woods, such as dry evergreen wood, burn fast and produce sparks, but often this is all you have. Dry aspen, dry alders, and maple tree limbs all make very good wood that will last for hours. A fire will burn overnight if you lay two green logs across the burning campfire so that flames rise between them. If they get a good start before the rest of the dry wood burns up, they will smolder all night.

When it is difficult to get a fire burning, be sure it doesn't go out while you are sleeping or during a rainstorm. Always keep at least one coal alive. At night bank the fire first with ashes and then a layer of dirt so the coals will stay alive. If it rains, cover the banked fire with bark, a flat stone, or whatever waterproof covering is at hand. When you move, carry a live coal in a tin can or bark container. Cover the coal with a 1-inch-thick layer of ashes, and it will not burn the container or die for as long as forty-eight hours. Rotten but dry wood also will hold a fire for a long time without bursting into flame. It can be carried along and blown into flame when needed.

How to Find the Right Direction

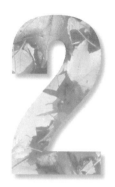

Last year near a small town in upper Michigan, a couple stopped at a motel. It was early in the afternoon and the elderly lady decided to go for a walk. She never returned. Weeks later a search party found her body beside a wooded road about 12 miles from the motel.

Even though it was summer, hypothermia set in after dark and she expired. Yet if she had known the right direction, she could have walked to help in a half hour.

We live on the edge of a large expanse of forest, and several times lost deer hunters have followed the light to our cabin after they got lost. Some are seasoned outdoorspeople. Most times they have no idea where their vehicle is, and even after I find it for them, they are so disoriented they don't know the way back to town until I tell them. Usually they are on the verge of exhaustion, and in the Wisconsin northwoods in winter, an exhausted human might not last until morning.

I get turned around about as often as anyone, and always have. But because I know I have this weakness, I have trained myself to react wisely when I discover I am not walking in the right direction. One good example happened during a western hunting trip.

I was tracking an elk on a mountainside near Pinedale, Wyoming, when I finally lost track of the herd. Then I realized that the peak I had absently been looking at for some time was not the peak I thought it was.

I remember feeling in my pocket for the compass and the great feeling of utter joy and relief that came over me when my groping fingers touched it. With compass in hand, I plotted a course. At first I

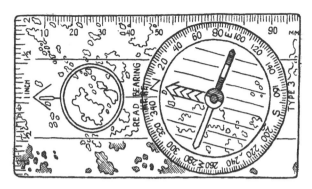

Figure 6
....

Every outdoorsperson should know the basic fundamentals of using a compass.

was tempted to walk due north, hoping to hit the horse trail. But I changed my mind when I realized how easy it would be to walk right beside the trail and never know it was there. I decided instead to walk east to a large burned-over area, follow its edge to the north side of the peak, and then walk west to the horse trail.

I had barely started walking when it began snowing heavily, almost blotting out the landscape. With no sun to guide me, the compass literally became a life-saving device. At that I didn't reach the trail until just before dark. I could have easily died on that peak that night, because after it stopped snowing it turned bitterly cold. The compass literally saved me.

No one should set out into unfamiliar territory without a compass (Figure 6). However, if you happen to be stranded in a polar region or in an exceptionally ore-rich territory where compasses don't work properly, or if your compass is lost or damaged, there are still several ways of determining the proper direction.

First, as most everyone knows, the sun rises in the east and sets in the west. But it neither rises in a due east direction or sets in a true west direction except in certain areas. In fact, in the far north the position of the sun can be very misleading, and so the stick-and-shadow method (Figure 7) should be used to plot due east and west. Furthermore the stick-and-shadow method can sometimes be used on

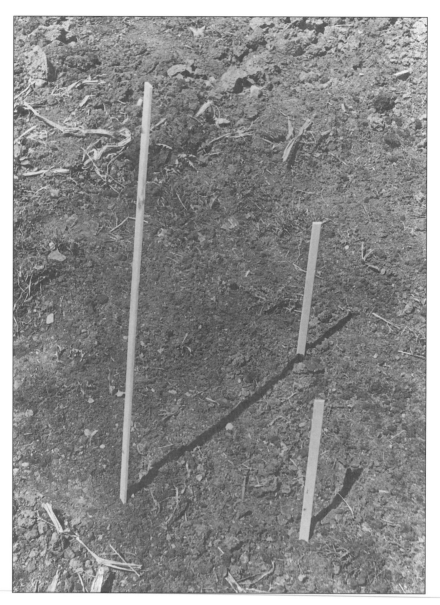

Figure 7

Shadow sticks used for finding directions. Using the longer stick's shadow, the shorter sticks lie east and west of each other when placed in the ground ½ hour apart.

cloudy days when the sun isn't visible because even on a cloudy day the sun might cast a shadow. (The moon also can be used if it is bright enough to cast a shadow.)

First cut a stick at least 3 feet long and stick it upright in the ground where the ground is flat and bare of vegetation. Then cut two marker sticks, each about 1 foot long, and stick one in the ground at the tip of the shadow cast by the 3-foot stick. About ½ hour later drive the second stick into the ground at the tip of the shadow again. It will have moved from the first mark. Now cut a direction pointer stick, sharpen one end, and lay it against the two marker sticks with the sharp end against the second marker stick. The sharpened end will point east and the blunt end will point west. This will be true anywhere in the world, since the sun always moves in an east to west path.

Now having marked true east and west, align your body with the direction stick so your extended right arm will point east and your left arm directly west. Now you will be facing north. With all four directions found, you can plot your travel path from them.

A watch or clock can be used to indicate directions when the sun is shining (Figure 8). Point the hour hand at the sun. Halfway between the hour hand and twelve o'clock will be south. If the sun isn't clearly visible, place a stick match vertically on the center of the watch face to see if it will cast a shadow. If it does, align the shadow with the hour hand. Halfway between the shadow and twelve o'clock will be roughly north.

Actually, shadows from natural objects roughly indicate directions whenever you know the approximate time. In early morning, they should lay nearly west; at mid-morning, northwest; at noon, north; mid-afternoon, northeast; and at sunset, east.

At night if the moon isn't shining enough to cast a shadow, and the stars are visible, find the North Star to determine north direction. This star is always located in the same position in the sky, at the end of the handle of the Little Dipper. For practical purposes the entire constellation Little Dipper is close enough to true north for short journeys, when there is no pinpoint destination in mind.

Actually any bright star can be used for plotting directions: Drive a stick in the ground and then back off about 10 feet and drive another in the ground so you can sight across the top of the two sticks at the star (see Figure 9). If you watch the star for several minutes across the tops of the stick, it will either rise, fall, or swing to the left or to the right. If it falls you are looking west, if it is rising you are sighted toward the east. If it swings toward the left you are looking north.

Survival

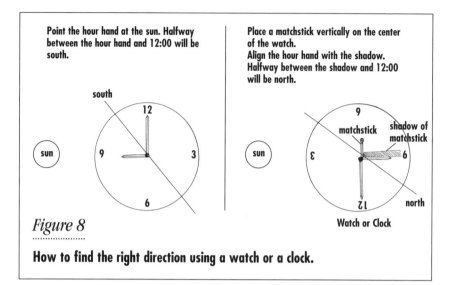

Point the hour hand at the sun. Halfway between the hour hand and 12:00 will be south.

south

12
sun 9   3
6

Place a matchstick vertically on the center of the watch.
Align the hour hand with the shadow. Halfway between the shadow and 12:00 will be north.

9
matchstick   shadow of matchstick
sun   ε   9
Zl   north

Watch or Clock

Figure 8

How to find the right direction using a watch or a clock.

Swinging toward the right indicates south. But you only have to remember that a rising star indicates east, and a star moving toward your left hand will indicate you are sighting across the sticks in a northerly direction, since the other two directions are opposite.

After you find the right direction to travel, by the position of the sun, stars, or moon, study the vegetation and topography to see if they contain clues to the four directions. Then, if the next travel day is cloudy, take your clues from the surrounding habitat. In many regions the prevailing westerly winds will shape shrubs and small trees so they lean in an easterly direction. Watersheds will follow a certain direction, and rivers and major streams will flow in one direction. Sand dunes and snowdrifts will be shaped by the prevailing winds into repetitive patterns that will indicate directions.

South slopes will probably have different vegetation than north slopes. Lakes and ponds or clearing also can provide clues if they are ringed by deciduous trees. The trees on the north side of the opening receive more sunshine, leaf out first, and consequently drop their leaves earlier than trees on the other three sides. Closely observe the green plants. Some indicate directions. The compass goldenrod (*Solidage nemoralis*) puts forth a brilliant flower that usually points north. The rosinweed (*Silphium laciniatum*) flowering head faces east and does not follow the sun. Prairie dock (*Silphium terebinthinaceum*) and prickly lettuce (*Lactuca scariola*) both have leaves that point north and south.

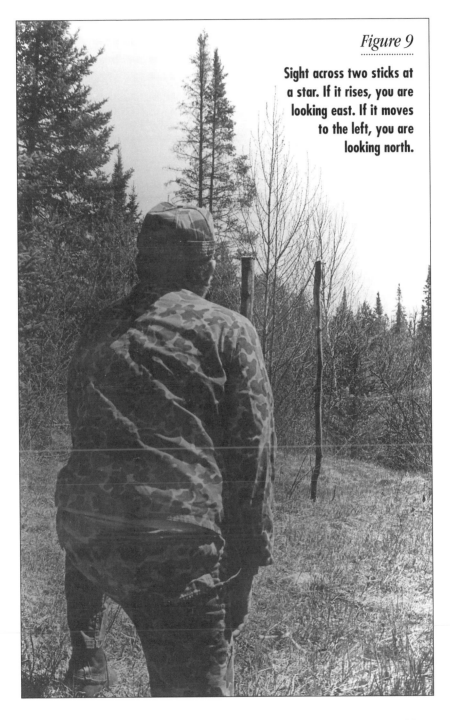

Figure 9

Sight across two sticks at a star. If it rises, you are looking east. If it moves to the left, you are looking north.

All of these methods of finding the directions should be practiced and committed to memory before an emergency develops. Then they will be second nature.

Let's set up a scenario that could easily occur to hunters, anglers, photographers, or sight-seers who contract a light plant to fly them over remote territory. The plane is forced to crash land and the pilot is killed. Your are on your own. After a few hours the shock of the accident will wear off, and you will start to think about getting out on your own. A flight plan was not filed, therefore a search party might not be initiated for several days. Thinking back over the journey, you remember seeing a highway out the right window. The sun was shining into the airplane from the left-hand side. The time was about noon.

At noon the sun is in the southern sky, therefore the highway must lie to the north since it was visible in the opposite direction. Now you know you will have to walk in a northern direction to get out, but cloudy weather has set in, and you don't have a compass. You think you know which direction is north, but you're not sure. You wisely decide to wait until the sky clears so you can tell directions. Finally about an hour after dark, the clouds roll back and the stars are visible. In the brief time that the sky is clear, you spot the Little Dipper, and realize that if you walk toward the Little Dipper, you will be walking toward the highway. You prudently decide to wait until daylight to start walking, and so you don't forget which direction you were looking when you spotted the Little Dipper, you create a marker pointing toward it. This marker can be a long stick, a line of stones, or even an arrow drawn in the dirt or snow. Next morning you set out, and by aligning trees and other natural objects, you continue to walk in a straight line. In six hours you stumble onto the highway and help soon arrives.

Finding Water

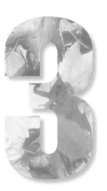

ater is easy to find on most of the remote places left on earth. The far north has snow and ice in winter and plenty of surface water in summer. Jungles are well watered, and many plains areas have rivers and potholes full of water.

Most of this surface water is contaminated and should be treated or boiled before it is ingested. Be sure to take water purifying tablets along if you will be flying over or traveling through remote areas. But if you don't have tablets, the water should be boiled at least ten minutes before being consumed. Only in a dire emergency should untreated surface water be consumed, and then a doctor should be advised after you reach civilization again.

Desert and arid regions are a different matter. In the desert dying of thirst is a distinct possibility, and every desert traveler should develop their water finding skills before going into one.

A person in the desert who did not exert him- or herself could live from two to three days with temperatures 100 degrees or more without water. At 50 to 75 degrees a person can live up to ten days without water. In the desert an inactive person can live for five days if he or she has two quarts of water per day. On the same amount of water at 75 degrees, the same person should live ten days. In cool temperatures a person can be mildly active and live on two quarts per day indefinitely.

Fortunately water is found nearly everywhere; even on the driest desert, it sometimes can be located. If such dire emergency arose that you would have to try to walk out from the desert without water and without a particular destination in mind, head for the roughest ground or for visible vegetation. If you can get to hills, there might be water near their base. A dry creek bed also might have water some-where running underground. Palm trees, cattails, grass, bushes, and greasewood can grow only where water is found near the surface. Animal trails probably lead to water in the desert. Birds also can point out a waterhole. They often circle over a water source, or their flight patterns are often directly toward water. Animals might scratch at the surface where water is close to the surface, and sometimes honey bees or other insects will gather on moist ground.

If you have a piece of plastic along on your person, or in a strand-ed vehicle or airplane, a solar still can be made (see Figure 10). Dig a pit in the lowest land available, about 2 feet deep and 3 feet in diame-ter, or as large as your sheet of plastic will cover. Leave enough slack so that you can place a rock in the center of the plastic to pull it down to a cone shape. But the first step after digging the pit is to place a tin can, a shoe or hat, or another object that will hold water at the center of the bowl. Now place the plastic across the top of the pit and hold it around the rim with sand or rock. If the ground around the pit holds any moisture, it will evaporate out and condense on the plastic. Then it will run down the sides of the cone to drip into the container under the plastic.

Up to three pints of water per day can be extracted from some desert soils this way. Try to remove the plastic only once per day, just before dark. If any other source of moisture is available, even the pulp, stems, or leaves from plants, it can be placed under the plastic. The plant juice will evaporate and condense again into water also. A solar still can be used to convert swamp or alkali water, or even the solution from the radiator of a disabled vehicle, to pure drinking water. Dig a trench under the plastic and fill it with the contaminated water.

Don't forget you can also recycle your own urine in this way.

When water is available, conserve it as much as possible by mov-ing only during the coolest part of the day. Talk very little and don't smoke or eat unless your food is full of moisture. Breathe through the nose and keep your clothing on because this will cut down the rate of perspiration somewhat. When you rest in the shade, try to make a bed about 1 foot above the sand. It can be 30 degrees cooler a foot above the ground. If you can't rest above the ground, dig down into the sand about 2 feet.

The human body can store water for short periods to some extent. Drink all the water you can before you set out on an arid journey. It is possible to saturate the tissues enough so that you can go a day or

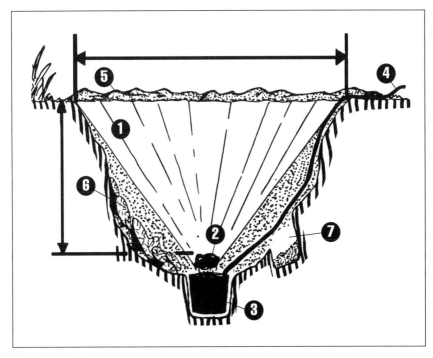

Figure 10

Desert Solar Still.

Legend:

1. Sheet of wettable plastic, 6-foot diameter.

2. Smooth, fist-sized rock for forming cone of plastic.

3. Pail, jar, can, or cone of soil, plastic, or canvas to catch water.

4. Drinking tube, ¼-inch plastic, about 5 feet long (desirable but not necessary).

5. Soil to weight plastic sheet and seal space. A good closure is important.

6. Line hole with broken cacti or other succulents.

7. If nonpotable water is available, dig a soaking trough around inside of hole. Carefully fill the trough to prevent impure water from running down and contaminating the water-catching container.

two without serious dehydration. Some travelers place a pebble or two in their mouths to keep the saliva flowing so the mouth doesn't feel too dry.

Watch also for water holes built in extremely remote locations for desert sheep. They are called guzzlers. Also, if you are lucky, you might spot a windmill, or cattle or sheep watering pond.

The prickly pear cactus grows in great quantities and its pad and fruit both contain large amounts of juice. Try not to get scratched; its thorns are long and wicked. Also the stalks of mescal, sotol, Spanish bayonet, and barrel cactus can be cut and drained of their juices for emergency use. Cut the pulp into pieces and suck on them.

Collect rainwater in hollows in the ground coated with plastic or cloth. Sop up water from puddles with clothing or handkerchiefs. Quickly dam up any nearby trenches to form pools.

Dew can be heavy, even on the desert on occasion. It will collect on stones, vegetation, or metal surfaces, such as auto bodies or airplane wings. Mop it up with a cloth and squeeze it out into a container. If there are nearby trees, the dew collects on the surface of the leaves. Mop it up also. When tall grass or brush is wet with dew, tie rags around your ankles and walk through the dew soaked vegetation. Wring out the rags in a container afterward.

In arid regions where grass is growing and has been growing for many years atop rocks, there will be a layer of muck or mud below the grass. Dig into this muck to look for water. There might be water just underground. Dig out the earth filler in cracks and let the water run out.

In arid regions keep an eye out for cottonwood trees. Find the largest cottonwoods. They are almost a sure indicator of water. Dig in any nearby low places for water. White brush growth is also a sure indicator of water; mesquite growth probably indicates a dry area.

Anytime you can find nonpoisonous plants or trees with green leaves, you can use the plastic bags from your survival kit to create a "leaf still" that will supply drinking water (see Figure 11). Without cutting the leaves from the plant, loosely wind or tie as many as possible into a bunch. Aerate a plastic bag to expand it to a round shape. Then slide the bag over the bunch and adjust it so the plastic doesn't touch the leaves. Place a small clean pebble in the bag, tie it at the top, and shape the bag so the pebble creates a small reservoir at the bottom to collect the moisture.

When the sun starts shining, it will draw water vapor from the leaves. The vapor will suspend or condense in droplets on the inside

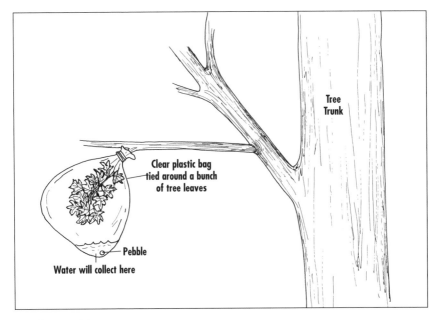

Tree Trunk

Clear plastic bag tied around a bunch of tree leaves

Pebble

Water will collect here

Figure 11

Leaf still.

of the bag. Eventually the moisture will condense into larger drops and trickle down the sides of the bag to the reservoir. Remove the bag carefully and extract the moisture. Don't leave it overnight without collecting the water, or its moisture might be reabsorbed into the leaves. A surprising amount of water can be collected this way, but create as many stills as you can to have a reliable source of water. The leaves in the bags will have to be changed each day.

You can extract water from cut leaves, water plants, pieces of cactus, or even damp soil with a "stump still" (Figure 12) made with a plastic bag. Place the leaves or plant pieces in the bottom of a bag and set it on a stump, rock, or earth mound. Use your "handy cloth," a T-shirt, or a few pairs of socks to create a trough inside the bag, which is around the outside of the stump. Tie the top of the bag so it is airtight and suspend it from a tree branch. The water that condenses will run down the sides of the plastic bag to be soaked up by the cloth. The cloth can be wrung out into a container, or the moisture sucked out directly into your mouth. The stump still can be left overnight without losing the collected water.

Survival   **21**

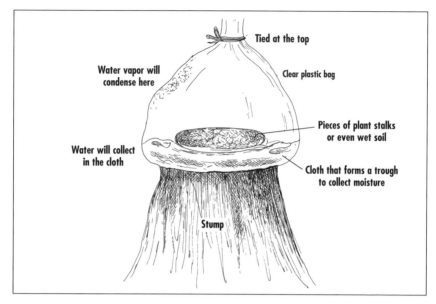

Tied at the top

Water vapor will
condense here

Clear plastic bag

Pieces of plant stalks
or even wet soil

Water will collect
in the cloth

Cloth that forms a trough
to collect moisture

Stump

Figure 12

Stump still.

Streams, rivers, and lakes flow in great profusion in most northern
and mountainous areas, and water usually can be found without
much trouble. If possible, it should be boiled for ten minutes. Water,
even in remote places, can be contaminated with a half dozen dis-
eases that are carried by animals. But if you can find a spring that
bubbles up from the ground, the water will probably be pure.

Stagnant water, even if it is badly contaminated with algae or mud,
can be made potable by straining it through a filter made by tying a
trouser leg at its bottom, partially filling the leg full of clean sand, and
then pouring the water into the leg so it must run through the sand.
Catch it in a container. It also should be boiled before drinking.
Several layers of cloth will also strain most particles of contamination
from the water, and sometimes you can dig a hole into the bank a few
yards inland from the shore of a pond and find water that is clean. It
also should be boiled if possible.

Sometimes a vessel can be hollowed out of wood, or a bowl-
shaped stone can be found that will hold enough water to boil. Of
course if you have no choice, drink the cleanest, coldest water you
can find.

It is possible that you will be caught along a seacoast in a survival situation without fresh water. Often water that is drinkable can be found back away from the seacoast by digging into the sand. If you don't dig too deeply, the slightly salty water is palatable. Dig mud holes to catch rain water.

Where snow and ice are present, no one will die of thirst. Eat snow if you can't melt it. Melt it only if you have a plentiful supply of fuel. It takes 10 inches of snow to make 1 inch of water. Eating snow and ice will not make your mouth sore if you only eat small amounts at one time.

Finding Food

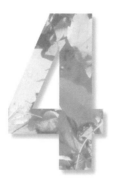

S tarving to death is not an immediate problem. Most of us can go weeks without eating if necessary. In fact, for many people, after about three days, the sensation of hunger leaves and doesn't return for a week or more. But food is an important morale builder, as well as fuel for the muscles and brain, and as soon as adequate shelter is constructed most people will start looking for sustenance.

If you are stranded along a watercourse, look for clams, crayfish, and fish. Fish can be caught by hook and line, speared, or caught in traps. Fish hooks can be fashioned from twigs, fish skeletons, small animal bones, or thorns (see Figure 13). A gorge-type fish hook can be made by just sharpening a small twig on each end. Make a groove at the center for fastening the line.

Fishing line is somewhat harder to obtain. Some clothing can be unraveled enough to produce a fish line. A leather belt can be cut into thin laces and used for fishing line, and the inner bark of some trees, when cut into strips and knotted together, is strong enough to make fishing line. Wire from a vehicle or airplane also might be used for line.

A fish spear (Figure 14) can be made from forest materials. We made spears for spearing suckers when I was young by just cutting a green hardwood sapling about 8 feet long and 2 inches in diameter. Cut a V notch on the lowest end and sharpen both points very well. Barbs are not necessary on a survival-type fish spear, because the fish is speared and then held to the bottom of the lake until you can reach down and grab it with your hands. A crotched stick (Figure 14) also can be used to pin fish to the bottom where the bottom is firm.

After the spear is made, position yourself on a rock or log overlooking the shallows and stay as still as possible. When a fish comes

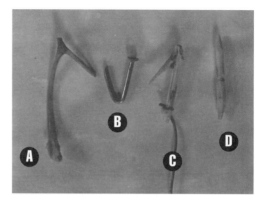

Figure 13

Fish hooks can be made of many different materials:

(A) Bird bones carved into fish hook shape.

(B) A nail.

(C) Fish hook made from a thorn.

(D) Gorge made from a branch.

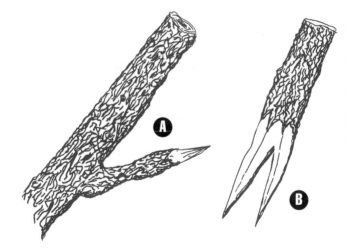

Figure 14

(A) Crotched stick.

(B) carved hand spear.

into view, slowly slide the spear into the water. Get as close to the fish as you can without actually touching it. Aim low to allow for refraction of the water, and then made a hard thrust.

If you've made a torch, try night spearing. Some fish are actually attracted to light, and others just ignore it. At night they are often in shallow water feeding and offer good targets. Fish also can be clubbed or killed by dropping stones on them when they are in very shallow water.

Be sure to put out a few fish traps also (see Figure 15). The traps can be made from rocks or with stakes pounded into the bottom of the lake. The shallow water section of a shoreline point is a good location for the traps, as is the inlet or outlet from the lake. These traps work well in streams also. Sometimes fish can be driven downstream into a trap.

Minnows are abundant in most lakes, streams, and rivers. Often they will supply more pounds of food than larger fish because they are

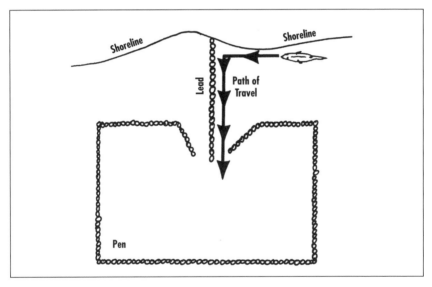

Figure 15

Fish move along the shoreline after dark. When they encounter the lead, they turn toward deep water and are confined in the pen. Use logs or stones for the lead and pen. They have to project above the waterline. The lead should be about 10 feet long, if possible. Build the pen as large as you can make it.

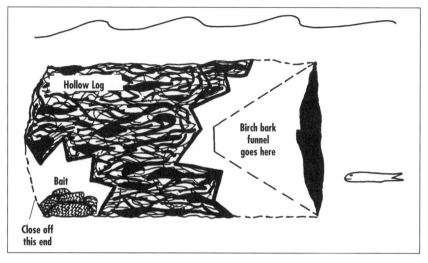

Figure 16
....

A minnow and small fish trap.

much easier to get. Make a minnow trap (Figure 16) by finding a hollow driftwood log, 1 to 3 feet long. Close off one end with branches or rocks. Then put fish guts or other bait in the end of the log nearest the branches. Place the log where you have seen minnows in the shallows and weight it down with rocks so that it sinks. Then find a birch tree or other type of tree with peelable bark and remove a section about 15 inches x 20 inches and roll it into a funnel. The small end of the funnel should be about 2 inches in diameter. Push the funnel into the log with the small end inward. A few such traps placed in good locations can catch two to ten pounds of minnow a day.

Minnows may also be caught with a net from a jacket (see Figure 17).

Strip the waste matter from their intestines by squeezing them, and then swallow them whole. They can be eaten raw or baked on a hot rock.

You can snare larger fish if you have some light wire or string along. Make a noose in the line, and when you see a resting fish, approach it very carefully and work the noose over its head, back of the gills. Then jerk it quickly.

Some fish can be grabbed by hand if you move slowly enough until your hand is under the belly. Then throw the fish out on the bank or grab it in the gills.

Survival   **27**

Figure 17

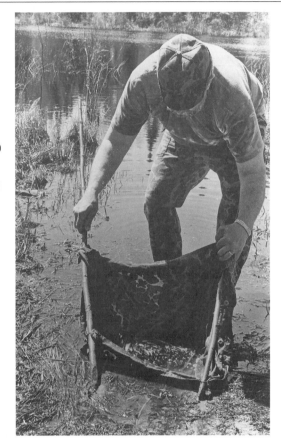

Pounds of minnows can be caught in one scoop with a net from a jacket. Minnows can keep you from starving to death when big fish are hard to catch.

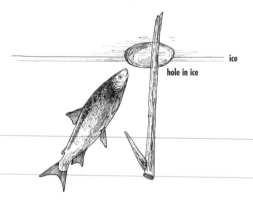

ice

hole in ice

Figure 18

Wooden fish gaff made from a tree branch.

Watch eagles and hawks also. Sometimes you might be able to scare them away from their kill of a large fish.

In winter chop a hole in the ice and make a sharp gaff (Figure 18) whittled from a tree branch to gig fish when they swim under the hole in the ice. Leave the gaff in the water until the fish is positioned directly above the hook. Then jerk it upward to drive the point of the gaff into the fish's belly. Keep lifting it to bring the fish up through the hole in the ice. A wooden gaff can also be used to catch fish from open water.

In many places rabbits and squirrels, along with gophers and chipmunks, porcupine, skunks, marmot, and other small animals, can be harvested by many different methods. Grouse, ducks, geese, crows, gulls, and all the birds of prey are edible, as are small songbirds.

Gophers and ground squirrels, tree squirrels, and cottontail rabbits can be found in ground burrows or in hollow trees. Where the ground is soft, you can dig the animals out with a sharp stick used as a shovel. If some means of carrying water is at hand, you can pour water down the burrow until you flood the animal out. If you want to reach the animal with a stick, use a twisting stick made from a forked tree branch. Push the stick against the animal and turn it to wind up the hair. Then pull the animal out where you can kill it with another club.

A snare (Figure 19) can be used to catch everything from a mouse to a moose, if the right sized wire is at hand. A snare is simply a length of wire, rope, cable, or even cord made of plant fibers that has been formed into a "hangman's noose" by tying a small loop in one end of the string and pushing the other end of the cord through it, forming a loop that will tighten up when pulled on. The loop is adjusted to the right size and set in an animal's trail, so that when it walks down the trail it will push its head through the loop, but it won't be able to get its legs and body through. As it continues to advance, the loop will tighten up and strangle the animal or tighten around its body and detain it until the survivor arrives.

Most snares are set to catch cottontail rabbits or snowshoe hares. These animals are abundant in almost every environment and have regular travel routes that can be noticed easily when there is snow, but also can be found in summer by looking for narrow trails through underbrush or berry patches. The snare is usually set where the trail passes between two saplings or other natural restrictions that will guide the animal into the snare. Also the snare must be secured to a substantial sapling or other anchor to hold the animal after it is

Survival

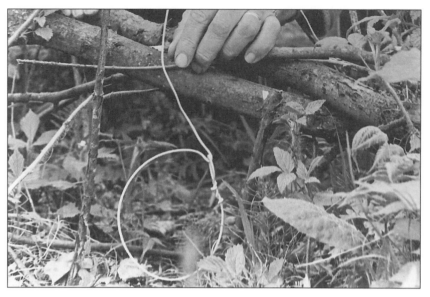

Figure 19

If you have the material, make up from forty to one hundred snares to set around your camp. It will require this many to keep you in food, especially during summer when animals do not follow trails most of the time.

caught. Jackrabbits are found on the plains or in some deserts. They do not follow trails as much as the other species, but they can be caught in snares placed where they follow animal trails along dry ditches or to waterholes.

Big game can be snared, also, if stout wire or cable is available. In remote areas of Wisconsin, backwoods folk snared hundreds of white-tail deer with barbed wire fencing a few decades back. They followed a deer trail until it passed between two closely spaced trees. Then they placed a log between the trees so the animal had to duck its head to pass under it. Next they formed a snare from the wire and located the loop of the snare so the deer's head ducking under the cross log would enter the snare. You can adapt this method to catch small moose, small elk, antelope, or caribou. In arid regions snares should be set near waterholes in places where animals are guided to a specific location by natural vegetation or topography.

You can also snare birds and animals by pulling on a noose when they are in the right position. Prop up the snare, attach a long cord, and conceal yourself nearby. When the animal or bird is in the right position, pull the cord tight.

Make a box trap (Figure 20) from forest materials. The trap is made so that when the animal enters to get the bait, a door will fall down behind it and confine it to the box.

A box trap can be made of logs or stakes. Cut stakes about 18 inches long and sharpen them at one end. Drive them into the ground about an inch apart to form a rectangle 10 inches wide and 18 inches long. Close off one end and roof the tops with a log or with several smaller poles tied to the sidewalls.

Fit the open end with a door made from materials at the site. The door must slide up and down in the four end stakes of the sidewalls. Tie a string to the top of the door and run it to the back of the trap. Fit this end with a trigger that will hold the door up when the string is tight, but drop it when the animal bites on the bait.

Finding bait for the trap can be difficult. Small animals usually have

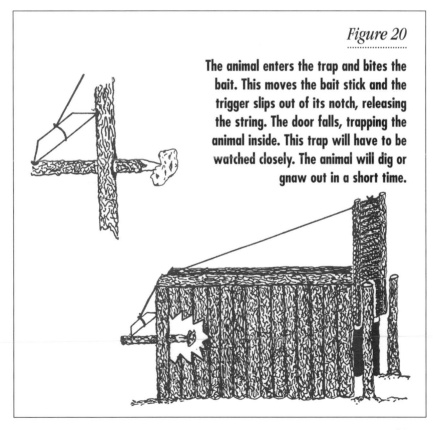

Figure 20

The animal enters the trap and bites the bait. This moves the bait stick and the trigger slips out of its notch, releasing the string. The door falls, trapping the animal inside. This trap will have to be watched closely. The animal will dig or gnaw out in a short time.

plenty of food, but they crave salt, and you can produce a salt bait from your own urine. First find a porous piece of wood small enough to be used as bait for a box trap. Place the piece of wood on a small bowl-shaped depression in a rock that will hold liquid. Urinate on this piece of wood so that the wood is soaking in urine. The salt in your urine will impregnate the wood, and after a few days, it will be salty enough to attract small animals. Fasten the piece of wood to the trigger of the trap.

If you are trying to survive in the forested regions of North America, look for a beaver pond. Beaver populations have exploded—their ponds dot almost all wilderness areas. One large beaver can feed a man for days. Moreover, their ponds will certainly contain fish, clams, crayfish, and frogs and might be a watering hole for nearby deer or moose, which also can be used for food.

You can get a beaver with a club. First look along the edges for signs of beaver cutting. If you see a tree that is partly cut off and the cutting looks like it is freshly made, the beaver will probably return to finish cutting it off that evening. Make a blind from tree branches or whatever is at hand and wait for the beaver to come out of the water. Be sure you are downwind of the animal and have a stout heavy club. Beaver have strong skulls and bodies, and it takes a tremendous wallop to disable one. Wait until it is clear of the water, get between it and the pond, and run it down. Beaver cannot move very fast on land.

If they won't come out on the bank, find the weakest part of the dam and pull it apart. A tremendous sluice of water will gush out. Stand by it with a club to kill any fish or muskrats that might ride this spillway out of the pond.

Long before the water is all out of the dam, the beaver will try to repair it. They will swim up to the hole in the dam and examine it, then disappear and return shortly with material to start fixing it. Hide nearby with a club or spear. If you don't get a beaver this way, wait until the water is low enough so that you can wade out to the beavers' lodge. Chase the beaver out by pushing a stick down into the lodge through the air hole opening in the top. When they come out, have a club or spear ready. They also might swim out to earth dens in the banks where you can dig them out. Beaver can be snared also if you have some stout wire along.

In the spring and early summer, the young beaver will not come out. But they will start mewing when the old ones leave. If you hear this sound, tear the lodge apart and get them. They will be at least as big as rabbits and are excellent eating. These methods are illegal in most states, but if your life is in danger, they must be used.

In the far north in the spring, look for a wetland where ducks and geese may be nesting. The eggs, young birds, and also the adult birds might be easy to get because you can catch the birds on the nest. Adult geese are respectable adversaries and could even break your arm unless you are armed with a stout club. They also can bite hard enough to draw blood.

When waterfowl are roosting in large flocks, you should be able to kill one or two by throwing a club into their midst. Also if you happen to find the waterfowl during the molting season, they cannot fly. They can be run down and dispatched.

In remote areas Franklin's grouse, spruce grouse, and ruffed grouse are unwary enough to allow you to get close enough to them to kill them with a club. In the spring watch on the ground at the base of a clump of willows or the base of a tree for grouse and ptarmigan nests. You might be able to get the hen and her eggs.

According to records would-be survivors have starved to death from what might be called "plate fright." They just couldn't eat what was available to them. Human beings can digest insects, snakes, lizards, grubs found under tree bark, and most other creatures that move about on the earth. Don't turn down any food in a survival situation. In early morning earthworms can sometimes be found on top of the ground. Squeeze them so they expel the contents of their innards and eat them raw or baked on a hot rock.

Don't forget the hundreds of edible green plants also. Most plants are edible, but a few are poisonous. Don't eat mushrooms or any plant with a milky sap; otherwise almost every other plant is edible, if not palatable. Even the buds and the inner bark from trees are edible, as are cattail roots, acorns, and cactus fruits.

Wherever you are likely to be stranded, there will be some species of pine growing. Most of them have edible inner bark, which is gathered by shaving away the outer bark and then scraping or carving the inner bark from the tree trunk or limbs. Eat it raw or roasted. In spring the new growth, which resembles a candle at the very end of the limbs, is edible on some species. If you can gather the mature but unopened cones, peel the scales away to find the pine seed at their base. The seeds of some species are edible, even tasty.

Cattails might be found in forests, plains, and even desert environments because they grow wherever areas of swampy wetlands are located. Cattails can furnish food all year around. In early spring the young cattails are growing up. Pull them up and eat the tender white base of the plants. Later in the season, early July in the upper

Midwest, the bloom spikes will be growing up. Near the top of the spike a miniature "ear of corn" grows. Eventually it will become the cattail, but at this point it will look like a pencil-sized green tube with a yellow center. Snap off these tubes, peel the husks away, and boil or roast them. They taste like corn on the cob. When they mature enough to bloom, pollen hangs thickly on the blossoms. It too is edible and will add a "corn" taste and attractive yellow color to flour or fish chowder. Gather it by shaking the blossoms over a container, such as a paper bag or a hat.

Cattail roots look like brown rope, and they seem to twine in every direction. They can be peeled, roasted, and eaten. At intervals along the roots, there will be new shoots growing. They are pure white and resemble a huge animal's tooth. Snap them off and eat them raw or cooked.

Cactus can furnish food also. If you can break open the stalk, the inner pulp of some species is edible, either raw or roasted. Furthermore, some bear fruits that are edible. In fact there are no poisonous cactus species. If you can reduce the cactus to food-sized bits; it can safely be eaten. To make sure you can safely consume cactus or any other plant, except mushrooms, follow this procedure:

First squeeze some juice onto the skin of your upper underarm. Wait ten minutes. If there is no reaction, taste a small amount without swallowing. Wait ten minutes. If there still is no reaction, eat a small amount and then wait five hours without eating or drinking anything to see if you have a digestive reaction. If you don't, it should be edible. If you do get a strong reaction, drink hot water to induce vomiting or swallow a paste of water and white wood ashes to neutralize the effects.

Practice finding and preparing edible wild plants and catching fish and animals before going out into the wild.

Making a Survival Camp

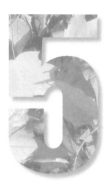

In all but a few instances the most self-serving procedure is to made a bivouac camp and stay put after you realize you are lost. Transportation is so rapid and search efforts are so intense and well executed in this modern age that it is nearly always senseless to move. Spend your energy improving camp, putting out signaling devices, and finding food.

If you can get a significant fire going and have a plentiful supply of fuel, a lean-to will usually be the best choice of shelter. With this combination you can withstand any temperature on the globe and be downright cozy in most situations. To build a lean-to, find two trees about 6 to 8 feet apart that have sturdy limbs about 6 feet above the ground. Remove all nearby limbs except one on the same side of each tree. Locate a sturdy sapling about 10 feet long and lay it across the limbs to form the ridgepole. Find at least six other 10-foot saplings and evenly space them at right angles to the ridge to form a roof. Weave flexible twigs or pine boughs among the roof poles to form a weather-tight roof (see Figure 21). If there is enough material at hand, close in the ends also. Build your fire about 6 feet from the front of the lean-to. As long as you can keep the fire going, this camp will be warm.

In the northern regions the evergreen trees are the best friend a lost person ever had. Their thick boughs can be used to make a warm comfortable bed and to cover a pole framework to make a shelter (see Figures 22 and 23). Moreover, the air temperature under a thick stand is actually up to ten degrees higher than in open areas. Furthermore, the thick tree evergreens usually breaks the wind, which considerably reduces the chill factor caused by moving air.

Therefore, if you are forced to spend the night in the woods in cold weather, by all means go into the thickest evergreen stand you

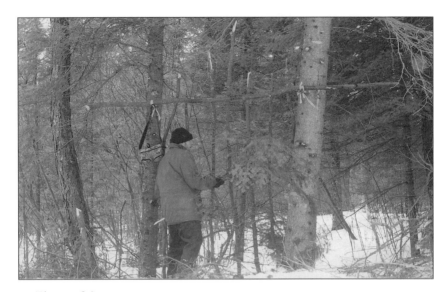

Figure 21

Building a lean-to shelter. Cut boughs and weave them between the roof poles to make a tight roof.

can find to make your survival camp. If you have a knife or hatchet the work will be much easier, but limbs can be broken by hand. Especially in cold weather, limbs will readily snap off.

There are downed trees in every forest. Find one that has been broken off a few feet above the ground but has not separated from the stump. Break off the branches on the underside of the trunk so that it will form a ridge pole. Leave the side branches attached and bring in the others to make a tent-shaped framework (Figure 24). Cover this framework with evergreen boughs woven tightly together, make a floor of evergreen boughs, and you have a dandy shelter that will withstand snow and wind. Also, put a 6-inch layer of pine boughs on the ground inside the shelter for a bed.

For a quick overnight tree shelter, look for a spruce or pine tree with limbs growing nearly to the ground. Break off the branches on the downwind side of the tree to make an opening large enough so you can sit with your back against the tree (see Figure 25). Weave the branches that you cut off into the other branches to make it even tighter than it is naturally.

Also, put a thick layer of boughs on the ground to sit on so that the moisture and cold from the ground will not reach your hips and

BASIC   ESSENTIALS

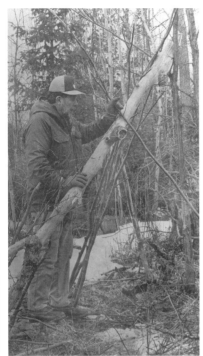

Figure 22

Build a pole and evergreen bough shelter starting with a downed tree. Such a shelter can be built without tools by breaking the branches off.

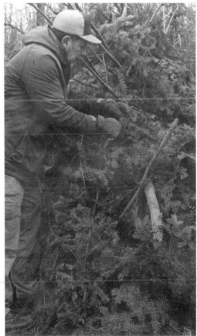

Figure 23

Cover a pole frame with pine boughs. When done with care, such a shelter can be made almost windproof.

Figure 24

A-frame shelter.

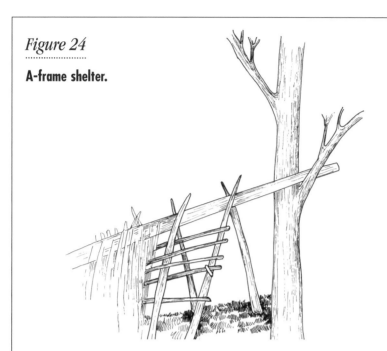

Figure 25

A tree shelter.

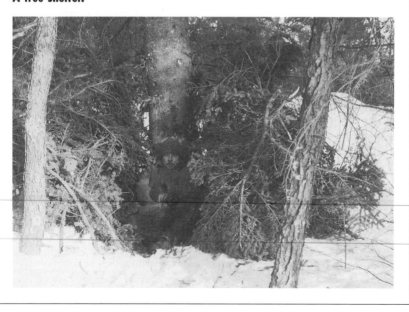

legs. You can rest fully clothed in such a shelter during the dark hours. Practice building these shelters before you get lost. Then it will be an automatic task.

In the plains or arctic regions you may get caught in open country with night coming on and a blizzard blowing up. Immediately look for whatever natural shelter is available. Find the lee side of a ridge, a gully, or the downwind side of a huge boulder, and make a shelter from the snow. Snow is usually hard packed by the wind in plain areas and can readily be utilized for a shelter (see Figure 26). Find a snowdrift at least 4 feet deep. They are usually located on the lee side of a huge rock, ridge, or stand of thick vegetation. Use your feet, a board, a forked stick, or whatever is at hand to create an opening in the snow. Collect sagebrush or whatever dry vegetation is at hand to create a lining to lie or sit on.

If you have your survival kit along, the tarp can be used for a roof and the plastic bags used to cover the ground to keep your clothing dry. Space blankets can be spread under and over your body to retain warmth.

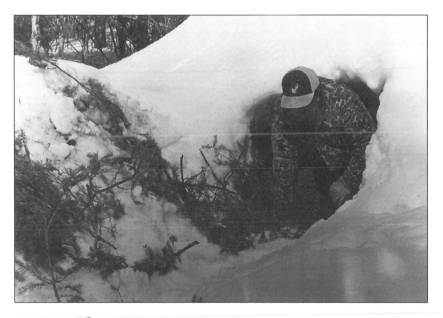

Figure 26

This shelter was hollowed out of a hard snow bank. It is also lined with evergreen branches.

Survival

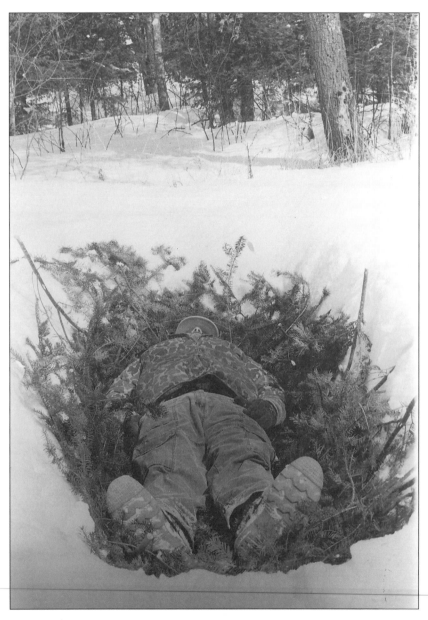

Figure 27

A trench shelter can keep you from freezing to death, but be careful not to work up a sweat making it.

BASIC ESSENTIALS

If no natural windbreak is available, make a trench shelter (see Figure 27) in the snow. I have made these shelters using just my feet for a digging tool. I make them about 8 feet long and 3 feet wide. They are formed at right angles to the wind so the sides of the trench break the wind. If grass, cattails, sage brush, or evergreen boughs are available to make a bed in the shelter, it will positively keep you from freezing to death. Also, if available, find enough vegetation to put a roof over the trench. Then the blowing snow will cover the top and make it even warmer. If you can't cover the top, push the snow you've removed from the trench into a ridge at least 6 feet upwind from the trench. This ridge will act as a snow fence and keep most of the drifting snow from blowing into the hole.

A large fallen log or rock pile can form one side of a survival shelter also. Lay poles on the log or rocks to form a lean-to roof. Cover the roof with evergreen boughs, grass, sagebrush, willow brush, weeds, or whatever is available. Make it only as large as needed. The smaller the shelter, the warmer it will be if no other heat is available except body heat.

Building a survival shelter is quite strenuous work, and it is easy to try to move so fast that you perspire heavily. This exertion can cause your body to chill badly when you finish and stop moving about. Discipline yourself to move slowly to prevent heavy perspiration, especially if you can't start a fire when you have finished.

If you are following a stream or river through the wilderness, keep an eye out for abandoned beaver lodges. Sometimes they are built far from the main channel because the area was flooded by the dam when the beaver built it. After the beaver have left and the dam has been washed out, the beaver house may be left high and dry. Enlarge the entrance so you can get in it, and it will form a completely tight and weatherproof shelter for sleeping. Abandoned beaver ponds invariably have a good stand of dead poles lying around. You can use them for shelter frames or for burning.

In plains areas sagebrush sometimes grows large and sturdy enough to use as materials for making a shelter. Usually the densest growth is in gullies and ravines. Here the sides of the gully will also help break the wind and make the shelter more snug. If the stalks of sagebrush are not sturdy enough to use for a frame, pile rocks or dirt clods to form a trench that you can sit or lie down in. Pile sage brush around and over it to make it more secure.

Look for a cave or overhanging bank in plains or mountainous or hilly terrain; it makes an excellent shelter, as does a partial cave if the sides can be covered with tree branches or other vegetation.

Although the Inuit lived in igloos in the harshest climate on the globe, igloos are not survival shelters. It is far quicker and easier just to burrow into a hard snow bank for the shelter than to make an igloo, unless you have the skill and tools.

A great many people are stranded in their cars each year during blizzards or because they get stuck in the sand or mud. Almost everybody who dies from such an incident left the vehicle and struck out on foot. Sometimes they had no clear idea of where they were going. It is far better to stay with your vehicle in nearly all instances. When it is cold, keep warm by running the engine periodically, but be sure the exhaust pipe is not plugged by snow or mud; also, keep a window open a crack so you won't be overcome by carbon monoxide poisoning.

If you run out of gas, you might keep warmer outside the car because the metal body of an automobile conducts heat away very rapidly. You will need a wind-tight shelter to survive very long in cold weather. Often there are materials or clothing in the car that can be used to make a lean-to type of shelter. Floor mats, seat covers, trunk liners, seats, and the hood or trunk doors can be removed and used as part of the shelter. You can make a warm bed by using the cushions from the front and rear seats. Cut each one open and remove most of the stuffing material. The hollow formed will fit the human body. The foam material you remove can be used to plug up drafty holes in the shelter. Nearby trees, brush, fence posts, or road signs can be used to make sides for a shelter. If you can survive for three or four days, help will surely arrive.

People have expired after their car became stuck in the sand in the desert. Usually they died of thirst and heat prostration after they left their vehicle and tried to walk out. It is far better to stay with the vehicle. Sleep inside the car at night and burrow under the car into the sand during the daytime. If you can't dig under a vehicle to escape the sun's rays, consider making a double-roofed shelter to rest in during the heat of the day. To do so find a natural depression or dig a trench about 2 feet deep, 3 feet wide and 8 feet long. Pile the sand nearby to use later. Roof over the trench with sticks, brush, plastic, or a tarp, if you have two tarps. Create a 12-inch-high sandbank around the edges of the roof and place a tarp over this to form a second roof. Conserve your water supply by not sweating. If you work on the vehicle to try to get it unstuck, do this at night, late afternoon, or early morning. Don't move anymore than you have to during the heat of the day.

You can use a large boulder, overhanging bank, dry streambed, or even the shady side of a cactus to shelter yourself from the sun. If you can't find shade, try to lay or sit on some object several inches above the sand because it will be as much as twenty degrees cooler than it is on the surface of the sand.

Small airplanes have been forced to land in the desert also. During the hot part of the day, the airplane will be too warm to stay in. However, the fuselage and wings will create shade, and this can be enhanced by using plastic or cloth material from the airplane draped over the wings to make a lean-to to turn away the sun's rays. Digging into the sand even in the shelter will help you stay cool. At night the interior of the airplane is an excellent shelter, in part because it will be safe from intrusion by poisonous snakes.

In cold climates the interior of the airplane is nearly the worst possible shelter because it will conduct heat away so rapidly. It will be mandatory to make a shelter outside the plane to avoid freezing to death.

Most airplanes that fly in the far north carry survival items along. A survival kit will usually include a tent or plastic tarp to use as a tent, space blankets, matches, flares, fish line and hooks, and dried food. You can use a parachute to make a lean-to shelter or as a ground cloth.

If you haven't any survival materials, fashion a shelter from the available natural materials as explained. The gasoline and oil and battery can be used to make a fire and for signaling.

Signaling For Help

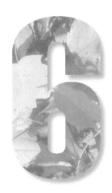

No one should go into remote territory without leaving word of where they are going and when they are expected back. If you walk out, leave a note in the vehicle when you are expected back. If you fly, be sure to file a flight report. Boaters also can leave word at a boat landing or with any available person.

Several devices are available for signaling in an emergency. A well-equipped survival kit will include a flare gun and flares, as well as a signaling mirror and whistle. Many survival kits also contain colored dye or colored cloth that can be laid out to make signals. Directions for using these devices are included with the kit, and there are further instructions in this chapter.

A cellular phone is an excellent addition to your survival equipment. If you have one along, and the phone is working, rescuers can be quickly alerted. They don't preclude the basic equipment and knowledge every backcountry traveler should have, though. For instance, even after being alerted, rescuers still might have to search for you, and physical signaling devices will be needed.

Furthermore, the batteries might be "numbed" by cold weather so they don't activate the transmitter, or the unit might be soaked from rain or by being dunked in a lake and won't transmit. Dirt might contaminate the device or it might be damaged from a fall.

Protect the phone by wrapping it in several layers of clothing placed inside a sealed plastic bag (if a commercial shockproof, waterproof container will add too much weight to your backpack). If the batteries are numbed by cold weather, place them next to your skin to warm them. In heavily forested areas or deep mountain valleys, the phone might not be able to transmit. You must then move to a clearing or to a hilltop. Do this before using up the battery power.

A great many people have been lost without any survival kit to aid them. They must improvise. Fire is the most noticeable signal that a survivor has at his disposal. The flame from fire is readily visible at night.

But be sure to build the fire where it can be seen: on an island, a lakeshore, a hilltop, in a large clearing, or even on a floating log or raft out in a lake.

Smoke can be seen for many miles in the daytime, and most of the forested regions of North America are watched over by rangers in fire-spotting towers or by regular flights of airplanes whenever the ground is snow free. A fire 6 feet in diameter, well smothered with green boughs, grass, or water plants will give off enough smoke to be spotted by fire spotters or searchers. Then help will arrive in a hurry.

If you can't keep a fire going continuously, lay the fire with tinder and fuel wood and cover it with birch bark, or whatever is available to keep it from getting damp. Then when you hear an airplane, light the fire. Three large fires spaced 100 feet apart in a triangular shape will signal an airplane that you need help.

Many times you can use an isolated, dead tree standing in a clearing or along a lakeshore as a signal tree. If the tree has dead branches so that it will burn well, pile grass, small dead branches, or dried moss in the bottom limbs and have it ready to set on fire. The flames will climb up the tree and make a torch visible for many miles. Again, the best time to light it is after you hear an aircraft.

Fire can be used to blacken a clearing, burn off a small island, or blacken tree trunks or rocks to make a signal to searchers. Anything you can do to the surroundings to indicate your presence will attract a search plane. After an airplane has spotted you, smoke will show the pilot in what direction the wind is blowing, so he or she will know how to approach the landing. If possible, have a landing site marked.

When you are signaling from a disabled plane or vehicle, don't forget that a tire will make very dark smoke when it burns. The oil from the engine also will give off dark smoke when it burns, as well as being a good fire starter. Gasoline is, of course, an excellent fire starter, but a spark can ignite the gasoline before it is needed. Tragic accidents have occurred when gasoline was thrown on a flame or on coals, so be careful. If you can mix the gasoline and oil together, it will be less hazardous for starting the fire and will burn longer after it starts.

Signal mirrors also can be contrived from the materials at hand. A piece of broken glass covered on one side with dark mud will make a usable mirror. A tin can lid can be polished until it is like a mirror, and a log slab kept wet from a nearby puddle can be used as a mirror to reflect light toward an overhead airplane (see Figure 28). In winter a slab of ice can be used for a mirror. Keep the mirror moving so that it will attract the pilot's attention.

When snow covers the ground, stamp out the letters SOS, filling in the letters with pine boughs or other dark materials. Make the letters at least 20 feet high if you can. Letters laid out in a general east-west pattern will cast a shadow and be much more visible from the air.

Pilots will fly low enough over lakes and rivers to look for tracks on sandbars. If you encounter sandbars, make tracks and figures in the sand as large as you can. Particularly scratch out SOS signals as large as you can make them.

If a tool is at hand to remove the bark from trees, peel several trees in a group because this will make an eye-catching signal from the

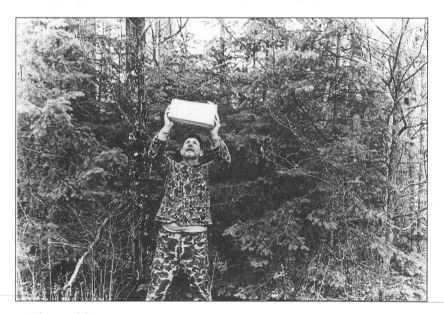

Figure 28

A piece of wood kept wet will reflect light and can be used for a signaling device. A piece of glass coated with mud on one side may be used in this way also.

land or air. Rocks or logs piled in the pattern of a cross will also attract attention. Make the cross about 20 to 30 feet long, if possible.

If you have some brightly colored clothing that can be spared, climb a tree and tie it in the top, where it will wave in the wind. Waving bright colored paper or clothing with your hands on the end of a stick (Figure 29) will also attract attention. At night torches waved around in the air are very noticeable.

Shooting also can attract attention if done at the right time. Wait until after dark when the hunting has ended for the day, then fire three evenly spaced shots. This is the universal distress signal. Then stay quiet and wait

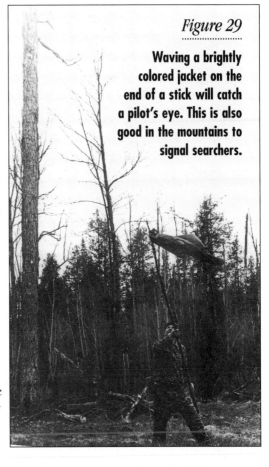

Figure 29

Waving a brightly colored jacket on the end of a stick will catch a pilot's eye. This is also good in the mountains to signal searchers.

for answering shots or shouts. If you get an answer, walk toward the sounds. But if you don't hear any more answers, and it looks like you can't walk out, stop and stay in one place until help arrives or until the next morning.

In deep wilderness shooting isn't likely to attract attention and it will only waste the ammunition you might need to get food. The exception would be if a search party was looking for you and was close enough that you would hear them.

Whistling can attract attention and can be kept up longer than shouting. A commercial whistle makes the most noise, but many people can "shepherd whistle" also. Do this by placing the thumb and forefinger together in the roof of the mouth. Then blow a quick puff of air. You will produce a sound almost as loud as a commercial whistle.

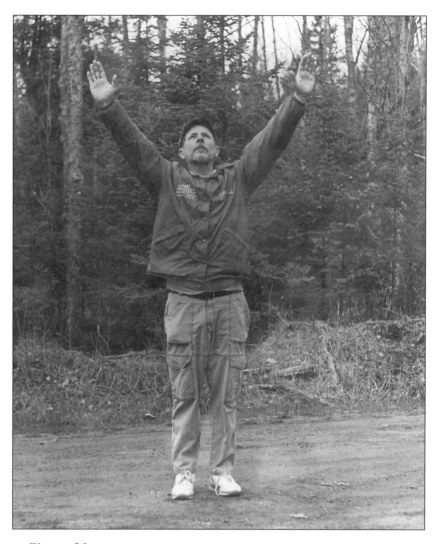

Figure 30

Be sure to learn this hand signal: It means "I need help." All pilots will recognize this signal. Do not just hold one hand up because that means "I don't need help."

BASIC ESSENTIALS

Pounding on a hollow log, a rock, or any metal object, of course, will make considerable noise, and this can be kept up for a long time to guide any nearby rescuers.

Signaling for help is largely a matter of common sense. Keep a clear head and utilize whatever materials are available. The first day or two that you are lost, sound signals will likely be the most effective. After that an aircraft search will likely be initiated. Then sight signals are most apt to be spotted.

Be sure to learn the hand signal for communicating with an airplane pilot that means "I need help." The distress or "I need help" signal is to hold both hands above your head (see Figure 30). Don't hold up just one hand because this means "I don't need help."

Above all keep a clear head, make your camp or trail as visible as possible, and make as much noise or create as many visual signals as possible. Do this and without a doubt you will soon be rescued.

Walking Out

Death, mental or physical illness, or just plain forgetfulness might result in your being stranded in a remote area without any means back home. Walking out might be mandatory.

But before you start walking, ask yourself a few questions: Are you physically able to walk out? Can you make snowshoes or fashion skis to get through the deep snow? Do you have adequate clothing? Can you withstand the insects? Can you find food or water? Do you know the way?

After you decide to walk out, take your time deciding what to take along. If you have a choice between taking a sleeping bag or shelter, take the shelter. You can sleep in your clothes. The tent will keep you from getting wet, which has possible fatal complications in cold weather.

Matches or some fire-starting device should not be overlooked. If candles can be found, they are excellent for starting fires along with fulfilling their intended task of giving off some light. By all means take along spare socks if available. Don't forget a knife or hatchet.

If no packsack is available, tie up the items in a piece of cloth or canvas and sling it over your shoulder like Depression-era hobos did (see Figure 31).

First locate a landmark before setting out. In heavily timbered country, this can be a faraway bluff, a lake, or an exceptionally large tree or rocky outcrop. It often is impossible to walk directly to a landmark. You may have to skirt swamps or go around lakes. To keep from getting off the trail, sight on some close-by object, such as a tree. Walk to it, then pick out another and walk to it. If this is done carefully, you will get back to your original route without losing track of it.

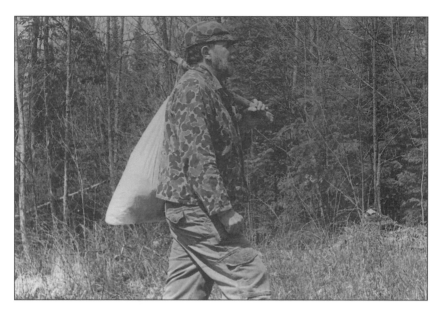

Figure 31

Carry your clothes over your shoulder tied to a stick.

When the sun is shining, of course, it will indicate the general direction. Walking directly into the rising sun will take you in an easterly direction, directly into the setting sun in a westerly direction. If you want to walk east during the middle of the day, the sun should be over your right shoulder; you're traveling a westerly route if the sun is over your left shoulder. When you walk south, the noonday sun will be shining in your face.

Night travel is an option in some areas. The insects might be so bad at night that you can't sleep and elect to travel. During the full or nearly full moon, this is quite possible even in wilderness territory. In the desert night might be the best time to travel to escape the hot sun.

The moon also rises in the east and sets in the west, so use it to determine your direction of travel. But actual travel routes will still have to be determined by lining up objects and walking to them. Most nights you can't see very far ahead and must use nearby landmarks. It would, of course, be very foolish to travel in strange, rugged territory on a dark night. When traveling at night, if you stop to rest, make a pointer to show where you came from and where you were going. Otherwise, the next morning you may have forgotten which tree or landmark you were walking toward or even in which direction you were going.

Of course no one should go into strange territory without a compass and at least a rudimentary idea of how to use it. Know also in which direction the broadest target is likely to be found. A road or large settlement would be a much wiser goal to aim at than an outpost, even though the outpost is much closer.

For instance, imagine that you are lost in the deep forest east of Red Lake, Ontario, Canada. You know that Highway 105 lies west and offers broad lines to strike out for. It is nearly 40 miles away and will probably take you five to eight days to reach because you will have to skirt numerous lakes. You also know that an outpost is located at Cat Lake only about 10 miles away, and another outpost is found at Slate Falls, about 15 miles distance. The outposts are closer, but if you miscalculate, you will be wandering in a huge expanse of trackless wilderness. Which should you choose? Without a second thought, strike out for Highway 105 directly west.

As mentioned in the signaling section, while you are walking out, try to stay ready to signal any airplane that might fly over. Airplanes

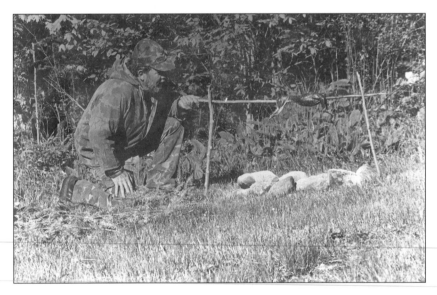

Figure 32

Stop early enough to make camp and cook food to keep up your strength.

BASIC ESSENTIALS

fly regularly in many remote areas and might see you if you are in an open spot ready to signal.

Once you start moving, resist the temptation to rush toward your objective. Walk at a moderate or slow pace and stop long before dark to make camp and cook food to keep up your strength (see Figure 32). Keep safety foremost in mind. Never step over anything you can walk around; never step on anything you can step over. Be extremely careful when crossing rivers and streams. If there isn't a safe crossing where you first encounter the river, follow it until you find one, or make a raft. If you encounter an extremely large lake or river, it is likely to be frequented by people sooner or later. Make camp and wait.

A river or chain of lakes is about the easiest route to follow in winter when frozen over. The snow cover is usually much less deep on ice than it is on the land, and it offers a definite highway that eventually will lead somewhere. But even in the far north, ice can be treacherous. Swiftly running water, unseen from the top, can cause the ice to be very thin over rapids or where the normal flow is compressed between two banks. A thick snow cover at the shoreline can insulate so well that the water doesn't freeze very thickly. Sometimes it is impossible to tell if ice is thick enough to be safe by looking at it.

But on the positive side, most ice in the north will hold up a person. You can usually tell if the ice is too thin by probing ahead of you with a sturdy stick. If you have a good knife along, lash it securely to a stick about 4 feet long and 2 inches thick. Keep jabbing the ice ahead of you as you walk. If the knife blade goes through, the ice is too thin to hold you up.

Some northwoods travelers carry a long, lightweight pole with them while walking on the ice. You hold the pole at the center so if you fall through, it will keep you from going down under the ice. But having participated in long treks over the ice, I know that after a day or two without any problems, most hikers will forget about the pole. It is too much trouble to carry. With no pole, your sheath knife is the best friend you have, because if you fall through in a place where it is too deep to touch bottom, you might not be able to get back up on the ice again unless you have a handhold.

If this happens, remove your sheath knife from its sheath very carefully so that you don't drop it. Your life might now depend on it. Grip it securely, hold yourself as far up on the ice as you can, and then drive the point of the knife into the ice. Use this as an anchor point to pull yourself back up on the surface of the ice.

If the weather is so cold that the snow is dry, roll immediately in the snow to remove as much water as you can from your clothing. Then get to shore and build a fire. If you can't build a fire, the only chance you have of surviving is to keep moving until your clothing dries out. Otherwise you will almost certainly die of hypothermia.

If you encounter a large river while walking out, follow the river. It will probably lead to help eventually. Moreover, you are very likely to encounter other people or see aircraft along a good sized river. Personally I would not try to walk any farther than the river unless I was sure that help was close by. I would either make a raft and float down it or make camp and stay put until someone came along. But like most other aspects of survival, this would be a judgment call.

Glaciers and large lake ice can have deep cracks filled with snow. If you fall in one, you might not get back out. About the only way to know if a snow-filled crack is in your path is to keep probing the snow ahead with a pole. If it is summer and the glacier ice is melting, water will be running everywhere, even making ditches too deep to cross. Travel from midnight to midmorning if possible to avoid most of the running water. Snowslides are also a hazard to travelers in the far north mountain or glacier terrain. If you get caught in a snowslide, try to swim to the top as if you were swimming in water.

In winter and fall the desert might be a friendly place to travel. The temperature is agreeable, and usually you can sight a distant landmark to keep oriented. A range of mountains in the distance, for instance, might be the only landmark you will need for days. The chief danger might be from flash floods or from the nights actually getting so cold that you will suffer from hypothermia. Try to rest in a cave or depression out of the wind but high enough so that a flash flood during the night will not catch you unaware.

Conversely, in the summer the desert becomes a hell hole, so hot and dry that without water a person can die trying to walk in the heat of the day. The best chance you have is to drink all the water you can, carry all that you can, and walk only during the cool part of the morning or late in the afternoon. The desert can be cooler after dark, but you might fall over a cliff or even walk in a circle without the sun to guide you. If you happen to have a flashlight, or if the moon is bright and you have a compass or trail to follow, night travel is an alternative.

Try not to walk in soft sand by traveling on ridges or troughs between dunes. Take good care of your feet by dumping sand out of your shoes regularly. If a sandstorm comes up, lie down with your back to the wind and cover your face with a handkerchief or other cloth. If you get caught out in the open in the heat of the sun, dig into the sand as far as you can and cover your body with sand. This can keep you twenty degrees cooler than the ambient temperature.

Snowshoes, sandshoes, or bog shoes can help a survivor stranded in deep snow, loose sand, or soft mud. They can make the bearing area of the foot large enough so it is possible to traverse otherwise impassable terrain. Pieces of board, sections of flat metal from an airplane, or several layers of cloth or canvas soaked in water and folded into a rectangle and allowed to freeze hard can make usable shoes. Tree limbs, driftwood, or small saplings are most apt to be used to make survival shoes.

Survival shoes (Figure 33) made like miniature ladders, about 1 foot wide and 3 or 4 feet long, will function as well as more elaborate designs and are easier to construct. Use approximately 2-inch diameter saplings for the side frames, with 1-inch diameter crosspieces. If dead but seasoned saplings are at hand, use them to save weight. Wire from your survival kit can be used for fastening the "rungs" to the side frames. If you don't have wire, consider strips of clothing,

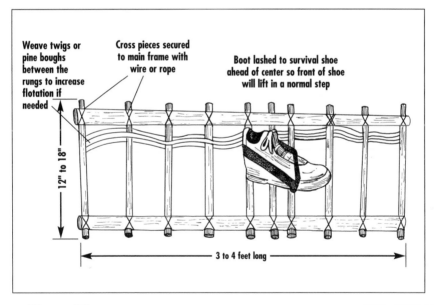

Figure 33

Survival shoes are for use in snow, primarily, but are also useful for traversing bogs or soft sand.

seat upholstery, leather laces cut from any spare boots, or even tree bark or roots. To increase flotation, weave twigs or pine boughs or even cloth or canvas between the cross pieces. The foot is lashed so the survival shoe will lift in a normal walking step. Lashings must be flexible, but strong. Possibly the best material you have along will be your bootlace. If you have to use them, then substitute strips of cloth or bark to lace up your boots.

For Novice Desert Travelers: Advice from a Desert Rat

If you are a novice to desert travel follow this advice, and you will never die of thirst or heat exhaustion in the desert. First, make sure someone knows where you are going and when you will return. Next, if feasible, take along a portable telephone or radio so you can report your emergency.

If you drive into remote areas in a vehicle, take along an extra spare tire, a spare fan belt, and a roll of duct tape for repairing radiator hoses. Watch your radiator temperature and stop to let it cool if it starts rising too much. Drive slowly and carefully to avoid hitting rocks, and don't cross creek beds or gullies without checking to see if the sand is too soft to drive on. Don't back off the roadway to turn around without checking for the same reason. Even so be sure you have jacks and blocks for raising the vehicle so you can get something solid under the wheels if you do get stuck in the sand. A portable come-along hoist and at least 50 feet of tow chain is well worth carrying. Next consider that, for whatever reason, if you get stranded you may not be rescued for up to three days. Besides a basic survival kit, have a shelter tarp, a sleeping bag, and five gallons of water for each person.

If you are hiking, imitate the desert creatures and only move during cool hours of the day. Try to take a portable telephone or a GPS unit. Never travel alone and make sure someone knows where you are going and when you are expected back. Have good up-to-date maps and study them beforehand to plan your route; if you do wander from the trail, know in what direction and how far you must travel to find water holes, ranch houses, or roads. Besides your survival gear, carry at least a gallon of water, and if you do get lost and find water, stay there until help arrives.

Getting Out by River

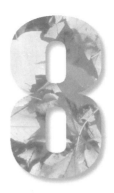

I f a river flows by your camp, you have a ready-made route to follow out. Every river flows to a place where help can be found. The river can be used as a carrier, so if possible make a raft.

Along almost every large stream or river, you will find material for building a log raft (Figure 34). Sometimes only two logs are needed to make a raft. Unless you are far upstream from an unnavigable part of the river, chances are the best thing you can do is make as comfortable a camp as possible and wait for someone to come along. This probably will not take long in most areas because people are floating and motoring on every large river during the ice-free months. Some rivers are as busy as highways.

In some places fallen but sound logs are strewn about in good numbers. Once you find the material for building the raft, reduce the logs to the right size. You will find that you need to use smaller logs due to the weight of larger ones. This can be done with fire if you don't have an ax or saw on hand. About the easiest way to build a raft is to lay the poles side by side and then lay another smaller log across and tie them together with rope. If you do not have rope, the logs can be held together with notched sticks.

Be sure to build the raft large enough to hold up everything you have as cargo. The bigger the better. Build the raft rectangular rather than square as it will be easier to steer. After tying the first layer of logs together, you will need to build a deck over them so that you can stay dry. Also you will have to find or make a pole or sweep in order to steer the raft. Travel using the raft only when it is light enough to see ahead. Even then stay close to the shoreline so you can land in a hurry if noise ahead indicates rapids or a gorge. Never enter unknown

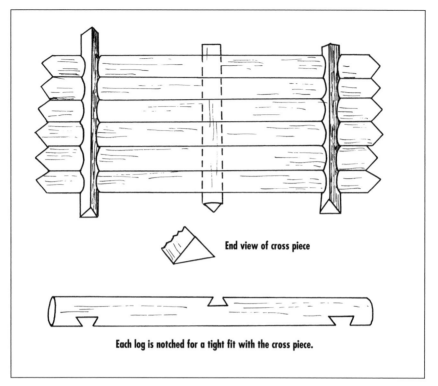

End view of cross piece

Each log is notched for a tight fit with the cross piece.

Figure 34

Making a raft.

rapids without getting out and walking ahead looking out for danger. Usually you can line the raft through rapids by letting it down on a rope. Another possibility is to take it apart and let it float down one log at a time. You can choose to build another below the dangerous area. Of course you could also take the chance of letting it float through, hoping it will make it, catching it below the rapids.

Usually it will be quicker and safer to walk out, rather than try to build a raft and float out. But there are clear exceptions: If you find a large stream or river with a good current but very little, if any, rapids or very shallow water, and you have more than 100 miles to go, then a raft might be feasible, especially if material for building one is close to the river.

Appendix 1
Surface-to-Air
Emergency Signals

T he traditional eighteen International Surface-to-Air Emergency Signals were often not well known to pilots. So they recently have been replaced with the following five easily memorized signals by the International Convention on Civil Aviation:

V   I require assistance.

X   I require medical assistance.

N   No.

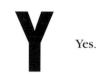 Yes.

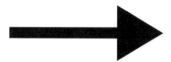 Proceeding in this direction.

Air-to-Ground Signals
consist of the following:

Will drop message: gun motor three times

Received message: rock plane, side to side

Affirmative: "nod" plane

Negative: "wag" plane

Fire or other location here: circle three times

Appendix 2

Basic Survival Gear

Most people know they shouldn't venture into a wilderness without suitable clothing. They should always wear sturdy boots, tough, tear-resistant clothing, and a suitable hat. Fortunately there are many suppliers of such clothing. Some suppliers of top quality leather outdoor boots are Rocky, Wolverine, Danner, Browning, Justin, and Cabelas. The Sorrel and LaCrosse companies make suitable winter weather boots with a leather top and rubber bottom. Winter weather boots should always have a removable liner so they can be dried between outings.

At present my favorite pair of leather outdoor boots is a pair of Rocky "Super Brutes." I wear blue jeans in summer, mostly wear Cabela's Camo clothing in fall and spring, and wool trousers in winter. My favorite outer jackets are made by Carhart and Browning. My favorite shirts are "stone washed" canvas in summer, fleece or wool in winter. These are available from Cabela's and WalMart, among others. I wear baseball style hats in summer and wool stocking caps, trooper, or fur hats in winter. Wool mittens and gloves or leather chopper mittens with liners are good cold weather choices, as are cotton socks in summer and wool socks in winter. I spend most of my time in the north woods, so these items are mostly tested in a cool climate. A knowledgeable desert traveler wear sturdy boots; lightweight, loose-fitting outer clothing; and a hat with a wide brim.

There are dozens of catalogs filled with dandy little products that you could find use for in a survival camp, but don't try to take too much. If a fanny pack weighs more than about two pounds, you probably won't carry it every time you walk out into the forest or desert, as you should. When making up your survival kit, keep in mind that, primarily, you need to drink, sleep, and keep from freezing or overheating in order to sustain life. You probably won't die without food or miscellaneous medical supplies before being rescued. There are many other items that will make a survival situation more tolerable, however. Here's what I carry in a fanny pack to sustain one person for *three* days:

Three-Day Pack

1. Two space blankets.

2. Four square feet of aluminum foil.

3. A plastic film canister containing fifty strike-anywhere matches.

4. A compass and a police whistle. I also have a pin-on compass.

5. Two clear plastic kitchen bags and two oversize leaf bags. Orange bags are more apt to be seen by rescuers.

6. A small, commercial first aid kit containing Band-Aids and Dristan tablets.

7. Water purification tablets.

8. A sturdy candle.

9. Small flashlight that uses AA batteries.

10. Two quarters, two dimes, and two nickels.

11. A lightweight knife with a 3-inch blade. I also always carry a pocketknife.

12. Insect repellent.

13. Orange marking tape.

14. A quart of water, but in the desert, at least a gallon.

15. Food is optional . . . if you don't mind the weight.

Use the space blankets to wrap up in or push both inside a large plastic bag to make a waterproof sleeping bag. The plastic bags will make a solar or leaf still, or serve as a ground cloth to sit or lay on, or an emergency raincoat or gear cover or to keep mosquitoes at bay. You can use the aluminum foil to make a signaling mirror, drinking cup, cooking pot, and numerous other items. Glue a piece of sandpaper inside the lid of the film canister to strike the matches on. Use the candle for light and for sustaining a fire long enough to start kindling. In addition to these fire starters, I have a magnesium fire starter and a canister of matches buttoned into each of my fall and winter jackets so I can't forget them. Turn one battery in the flashlight backward to prevent accidental discharge. The coins are for a pay phone if you encounter one. You can use the marking tape for making the trail to guide rescuers, and it can be used as rope for making shelters and has numerous other applications.

Make sure the knife is of good quality steel. My pocketknife is a Schrade, "Old Timer" series, and my daypack knife is a "Twistlock" by Cold Steel Company. Likewise, your compass must be absolutely reliable. My main compass is a "Sportsman" model by Michaels of Oregon. Other companies make reliable gear also, but stick to a well-known supplier. This is no place for cut-rate products.

Seven-Day Pack

A second pack, to sustain one person for a week or more, should contain, in addition to the three-day pack items:

16. A small aluminum cooking pot.

17. A week's supply of water purifier tablets or a PUR water purifier pump.

18. A spool of 40 nylon fish line, a packet of fish hooks, and a half dozen sinkers.

19. A signaling mirror.

20. A lightweight, bright blue down sleeping bag.

21. Enough freeze-dried food to supply 10,000 calories (five day's supply).

22. Nine square feet of aluminum foil.

23. Two Bic cigarette lighters, a packet of tinder made of 00 steel wool, interspersed with hemp rope fibers.

24. A hand-operated pencil sharpener, pencil, and small notepad.

25. A 10" x 10" section of 6 mm plastic tarp.

26. One-hundred feet of 32-gauge steel wire for rabbit and squirrel snares.

27. Twenty-five feet of quarter-inch nylon rope.

28. A folding camp saw.

29. An outdoor first-aid kit as listed in Appendix 3.

Use the fish line for tying components of a shelter together, repairing clothing, snaring and making traps, and fishing. Leave messages to guide rescuers on the paper. Use the tinder with the magnesium fire starter to create a flame. Tinder is meant to be used up first; keep the matches for later. Be sure to pull the steel wool fibers apart before striking the spark, and when it glows, blow hard to start a flame. You can make tinder with the hand-operated pencil sharpener faster and better than any knife. Find a dead, seasoned twig that will fit or can be shaved to fit and "sharpen" it.

The tarp can serve as a shelter, and the rope may be used for hanging the shelter or a dozen other tasks around the survival camp. The saw is for cutting poles for a shelter frame, cutting firewood, or clearing away vegetation to make a camp or a signaling icon.

Appendix 3
The Outdoor
First Aid Kit

S tate-of-the-art dressings, wound closure tapes, and
nonprescription medications allow the construction
of a very useful first aid kit for general outdoor
use.
Very often treatments can be improvised with other items on
hand, but prior planning and the inclusion of these items in your kit
will provide you with the best that modern medical science can offer.

Quantity	Item
2 pkg.	Coverstrip closures, 1/4" x 3" (3/pkg.)
1	Spenco 2nd Skin Dressing Kit
1	Bulb-irrigating syringe
5 pkg.	Nu-Gauze, high absorbent, sterile, two-ply, 3" x 3" pkg.
1	Surgipad, sterile, 8" x 10"
2	Elastomull, sterile roller gauze, 4" x 162"
2	Elastomull, sterile roller gauze, 2½" x 162"

10	Coverlet Bandage Strips, 1" x 3"
1	Tape, hypoallergenic, ½" x 10 yd
1	Hydrocortisone cream, .5%, 1 oz tube (allergic skin)
1	Triple antibiotic ointment, 1 oz tube (prevents infection)
1	Hibiclens Surgical Scrub, 4 oz (prevents infection)
1	Dibucaine ointment, 1%, 1 oz tube (local pain relief)
1	Tetrahydrozoline ophthalmic drops (eye irritation)
1	Starr Optic Drops, ½ oz bottle (ear pain, wax)
1	Micronazole Cream, 2%, ½ oz tube (fungal infection)
24	Actifed tablets (decongestant)
24	Mobigesic tablets (pain, fever, inflammation)
24	Meclizine 25 mg tab (nausea, motion sickness prevention)
2	Ammonia inhalants (stimulant)
24	Benadryl 25 mg cap (antihistamine)
10	Bisacodyl 5 mg (constipation)
25	Diasorb (diarrhea)
25	Dimacid (antacid)
2 pkg.	Q-Tips, sterile, two per package
1	Extractor kit (snake bite, sting, wound care)
6	1 oz vials for repackaging tablets, salves, or liquids
1	Over-pak container to make up a convenient kit

BASIC ESSENTIALS

Consideration should be given to a dental kit. Several are commercially available through backpacking and outdoor outfitters. As a minimum a small bottle of oil of cloves can serve as a topical toothache treatment, or you can carry a tube of toothache gel. A fever thermometer should be included on trips. People wearing contact lenses should carry a suction cup or rubber pincher device to aid in their removal.

Appendix 4
Ten Steps for Survival

1 Remove yourself from danger, such as vehicle explosions, precarious footing, or hazardous waterways.

2 Find a campsite and build a basic shelter.

3 Build a campfire. Besides providing warmth, a campfire has a calming effect and promotes confidence.

4 Find water. Treat all surface water or boil it for ten minutes.

5 Start signaling. Put out commercial signals, display bright cloth signals, and make tracks in the sand and mud and otherwise change the natural appearance of your surroundings so they will be noticeable from the air and land. Keep a smoky fire burning. Make all the noise you can. Keep flashing your signal mirror in all directions even if you don't hear or see help.

6 Look for edible plants. You can eat grass, cattail roots, insects, inner pine bark, berries, reindeer moss, plantain, violets, arrowhead roots, acorns, and most other plants. For safety, try very small amounts at first.

7 Try to catch fish or animals for food. Fish, clams, crayfish, frogs, minnows, rabbits, and rodents are most likely to be nearby. Set snares or construct traps for rabbits and rodents.

8 Move in seven days. If you're not rescued in a week, consider moving camp to a more visible location.

9 Find the four directions. Remember the sun rises in the east and sets in the west and so does the moon. Stick two three-foot-high sticks in the ground and sight across them at a star. If the star rises, you're looking east. If it moves to the left, you're looking north.

10 When it's time to start walking out, walk in a straight line by sighting on landmarks. In almost every region of North America you should find help within ten days. Go at a reasonable pace and stop early enough to make camp.

Index

BASIC ESSENTIALS

Survival

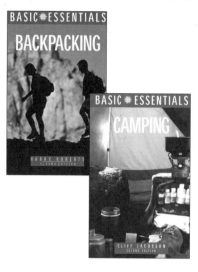
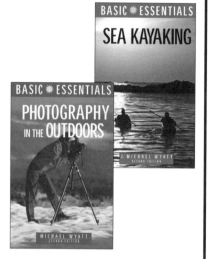